The Practice of Being

Anne Markham Bailey

Present Tense Media

The Practice of Being

The Power of Creative Awareness

Anne Markham Bailey

Present Tense Media / Birmingham, Alabama

ALSO BY ANNE MARKHAM BAILEY

Cold Stone, White Lily
Nancy Marguerite's Chopin
The Daring Egg

The Practice of Being

Copyright © 2021 by **Anne Markham Bailey**

All rights reserved. No part of this publication may be reproduced, distributed or transmitted in any form or by any means, without prior written permission.

Present Tense Media
4000 3rd Avenue S
Birmingham, AL 35222
www.presenttensemedia.com

Library of Congress Control Number: 2021917096

The Practice of Being/ Bailey, Anne Markham . -- 1st ed.

ISBN 9781733013895

Book Layout © 2021 Present Tense Media

CONTENTS

Foreword ix
Preface..xi
Introduction... xiii
How To Use This Book xix
Possibility.. 1
In The Beginning 3
Being Human 9
Longing 13
Waking Up 15
Union... 17
The Path 21
Awareness 25
Breath 29
Being the Body 33

The Journey of Practice 37
Practice Instruction 39
Becoming Intimate 43
Mental Weather 47
Wisdom 49
Choosing to Practice 51
Acknowledgments 53
Resources 55

Foreword

Words don't teach; experience does. This is something Anne Bailey understands. She also understands the power of words to bring people together and to provide road maps for personal and shared experiences. In this book, Anne does that with the skill of a master teacher and artist.

Anne and I met decades ago and a close friendship blossomed when we both began an in-depth study and practice of meditation. Anne dove more deeply than I. She attended solitary retreats in wooded cabins and monasteries, and she often spent weeks at a time in silent retreats devoted to nonstop practice from sunrise to bedtime. Without clinging to any one religious tradition or practice, she discovered their common denominator—what she calls "the practice of being."

If you are interested in understanding yourself, your purpose, or your world more fully, this book will be of value to you whether or not you have a religious affiliation or are an experienced meditator. All you need is a willingness to engage the practice—the simplest practice of all, so simple it may at first appear absurd, but if with curiosity you return to the practice again and again, as suggested by this lovely book, you will come to know its profundity.

The Practice of Being will not tell you what to believe or how to act; there is no set of rules to follow here. But you may find that the book calls you, as it did me, to question beliefs and patterns of behavior and to awaken the curiosity to look into the nature of *your* being, to recognize your being, to feel its presence, and to experience, if only momentarily, the very life source that we are.

This is where the road map of *The Practice of Being* leads, to a direct experience of the Source of Life, that which some call God. With the sensibility of a poet and storyteller, she offers the practice of being as more than a mere technique; she shows it to be a natural phenomenon—a human birthright—that promotes peace and joy in our personal lives and greater justice in our world.

Leisha Hultgren, Ph.D.

Preface

In response to my students' repeated requests for a practice book, I wrote this manual in 2019 and 2021, in a series of solitary retreats in Decorah, Iowa. The writing was accompanied by long walks, elaborate dreams, and deep sleep. I alternated the writing with drawing in the evening. My retreats coincided with the lilac blooms at Jamie and Bruce Adair's farm, a rare ground blizzard in subzero conditions, and the apple harvest.

Introduction

I learned to meditate in the Shambhala Buddhist community in my late 20's. I re-encountered key concepts that I'd first studied with WilliamTheodore de Bary at Columbia University as to why meditation is so important, the first being the possibility of attaining freedom from the suffering of cyclical re-birth as a sentient being. The second is the idea that one may realize compassion so pervasive that even if freed oneself, one remains in order to help free all other beings. Essentially the teaching is that you may get the carrot, and once you do, you're going to want give the carrot to your neighbor.

I was raised in the Episcopal Church in Mountain Brook, Alabama, and the essential teachings of Christ resonated in me at an early age. The Christ teachings on love radicalized me from the start. The church itself did not make as much sense. Then, as now, I was full of questions on all things human and otherwise. I lived in a world where the core Christ teachings on love were clearly not being implemented, yet few seemed concerned. As I encountered the brutality of systemic, psychological, and physical terror against Black people carried out by those who may well have been my parents' neighbors, I learned about hypocrisy. The *Life Magazine* images of the Vietnam War were blatant announcements that the core principals of love were not going to be practiced, particularly when the "neighbor" did not look like you. After many questions on my part and many tired responses from the priests, I left the Church after my confirmation at the age of 12. No one seemed to regret my departure.

I left Shambhala Buddhism as well, decades later. The stark contrast between what is preached and what is practiced was risen once again. Too many of the teachers in Shambhala sought and gained power and then abused students mentally, physically, and spiritually. Of course this is not a new story in religion. The reality crept upon me, a devoted student, bit by bit until I finally knew the truth in my gut. I needed to go. I gave up my community. I walked away from my context. I was confused and bruised. The loyal silence of my conformity prevented me from being able to talk with the people around me. I was cast as the one with the problem.

The idea that one can loosen and untie the knots that keep us separated from the freedom to manifest in our full glory is imbedded in my understanding of existence. As well, the view of an ultimate connectedness of all beings including humans, mollusks, hemlocks, stones, and air, appears to me as logical and provable. The third piece that shapes me profoundly is the power of practice as a tool for our transformation from the tyranny of mental fixation to the power of our self-existing creative awareness.

As a child my practice was being in nature. As a girl I came to art and to music. Later I found writing, singing, performing, sports, and study. I became a lover, a yogi, a mother, and a wife. I started psychotherapy. I lived in China, camped in Spain, became a poet and a book artist. I spoke French, Chinese, and Spanish. I needed money. I needed love. I suffered and could not seem to reach the core point of origination. What is the point of life, I wondered.

As I began to explore meditation, I also encountered the work of Mosha Feldenkrais, and for the first time as an adult, I felt my life as a body. Such discovery. This entry into being unfolded into a journey that is the heart of this book. Here we are on a planet that spins in outer space. We arrive out of deep time for what appears to be a brief journey on this planet's surface. What are we going to do? What really matters? Should we simply believe what we are told or rather explore for ourselves?

I'm an explorer. I have the good fortune of encountering teachers who have offered me the time, space, and context for exploring the great truths of existence.

Over my years as a teacher, Creative Awareness practice has evolved to awaken somatic or deep body awareness, mental pliancy, and deep connectedness as the essential creative state of being. This combination may well be love in its most fundamental form, the space that cradles our connections. My passion is to offer this material outside its traditional hierarchical context with the radical power of independent exploration as the primary key rather than the proscribed rules of engagement.

The well being of the planet depends upon our realization of connectedness, and from my point of view, exploratory practice such as Creative Awareness is what will bring us to an ultimate knowing based in feeling. As you come to feel the nuance and detail of your own being, you can feel me, the earth, the sky, the space where we unfold into being in our real power, in love.

Anne Markham Bailey
In the time of Covid
August 2021
Birmingham, Alabama

How To Use This Book

My deepest hope is that this little book can become a friend that encourages you to practice and to fall in love with your own practice of being. This is a small book that is easy to read, easy to hold, and easy to carry. I focus on a single practice that is simple to explain. The work is meant to be ingested in small bits.

Some parts of this practice book are thick; the sentences are long and the language is poetic. Other parts are instructive and straightforward. Both are written for your enjoyment. It is my wish that you might have access to the Creative Awareness practice that I have developed from my own many wisdom teachers across time.

This practice book is dedicated to the wisdom teachers who trained me to feel my own magnificent existence fully. Every aspect is included. Dark corners are included. Rage is included. Ignorance and brilliance are included. Our longing is the door, and the practice of being is the path that we take to manifest. I offer this to you.

{ 1 }

Possibility

The possibility of our lives is to create our own instruction manual, to construct the shapes, to sort the patterns of the people and places of becoming, and to become emboldened or perhaps simply curious, oh so very curious about the textures of being, to reach into the detail of our moments, intricate, ecstatic, and excruciating, to feel the breath as journey, to turn away, and then to return again and again.

From the ferry chugging through the blue-green water off the coast of Galway in Ireland, headed to the island of Inishbofin, I stood at the back of the boat and stared into the bright green wake as the water turned over and dropped back into darker blue. No wonder we suffer as we do, I thought. We're not taught how to be in this body once we arrive after birth. We're not taught how to feel fully. But we can learn. In the sharp wind on my face, I felt the shape of the practice in my life. I could see the repetitions in the waves moving onto the island shore, in the bowls of hot oatmeal that I'd served to my son in the morning as he grew up, as he stood with me on that boat on that day in Galway. I saw this practice book and the brilliant possibility of life that is ours to create, breath by breath.

＃ { 2 }

In The Beginning

Rage bursts the tight confines of my ideas about myself. A wind rises within and once aroused expands with heat, wraps into my heartbeat, gains momentum, acquires voice and stature. Once my rage suits up in all her finery, the flushed flesh and flamboyant phrase ready for an assault, I look for trouble amongst the ones I love the most. My rage is a storm reminiscent of the Alabama tornadoes strewn across my life, quick and devastating, a relentless path with no real target but rather a swirling roar in which places and people are lifted and tossed across the sky to fall flat and collapsed. What a hangover after, devastation assessed in silence, pieces gathered, shards swept in a quiet shame. Oh yes, I know about rage. Rage brought me to practice.

I wanted to live a life that I dreamed up. I was a young poet married to an artist friend from college at Columbia University in New York. We birthed a beautiful son called Edward. But our dreams differed and our life exploded. Fissures rose up. Alcoholism, new parenthood, my role as a nursing mother, the time off from my work as an MFA student, buried sexual trauma, our confusion as to how to live as artists and make enough money to survive – it was too much for us to handle. We separated. I fared poorly. I didn't eat. I had an affair. I attended to my son. My rage expanded into a numb and pervasive armor that I wore without respite. I couldn't escape the grief or the rage or the terrible sense that I'd simply missed the boat on my life, other than being Edward's mother.

A few years after my divorce, I attended a meditation seminar. I had met some Buddhist meditators at the Unitarian Church in Birmingham, and since my lover at the time encouraged me to learn to meditate, I signed up for a seminar that was held at a local non-profit. The meditators were seated on red cushions around the room on a red and white tile floor. The floor was patterned with the rise and fall of light and shadow through tall floor-to-ceiling windows. I sat with a pain in my shoulder and a desperation to achieve something, to get this right, to make up for lost time, to rise to the top and to fulfill the promise of my life. I wanted to escape the country and western tune sounding a closed loop in my head. I was on the verge of running away and never coming back to the ridiculous proposition of following the breath moment by moment. Were the organizers of the seminar in a cult? I wondered. My foot was asleep, so there was that to deal with. I wanted to be incredibly still, the most still, absolutely the most still and hence the most fantastic meditator of recent memory or perhaps ever. What dancing and celebrating there would be as I was lauded as such an incredible being. Oh yes.

But the matter of my foot was at hand. I was simply going to have to move it because of the unbearable feeling of needles that spread through my flesh plus the stabbing feeling in my back. Oh, it was a miserable state, being on this cushion in this absurd exercise that made me sleepy and irritable. If only we could just finish this session, if only I could just hear the ding of the gong so that I could get up and have a snack and some coffee. Perhaps that would set it right.

At various points, the instructions for the practice broke into my fantasies of enlightenment. I placed my attention on the feeling of the breath coming into my body, the moment when the air touched my nostrils and I pulled it in, past the sensitive hairs that serve as sentries in the nasal outpost. The air, as it passed into the cavity of the mouth, continues on its journey to the lungs. The lungs, ribs, and belly expand to make room for the outside world moving in and out. Another breath comes in, and this one is different. I can feel the left nostril more than the right.

While sitting on the cushion, I saw myself as a toddler, thoroughly pleased to be on my feet, taking steps towards my mother with her open arms, moving towards the encouragement and pleasure in her voice and in her eyes. In my mind's eye, she squats and calls to me as I move from foot to foot, pleased and safe and happy in this newly found upright motion after my months of practice, of rolling and rocking, exploring the physical being so recently acquired at my birth.

In this vivid memory, I hold my mother's eyes and her love fills my flesh. The love spreads to the boundaries and past the edges of my body as I sit on the cushion in the meditation hall. Tears roll down my cheeks. The dullness of sitting is pierced by this re-collected moment of first steps before doubt or fear were habitual and rampant. Warmth in my heart center opens to a simple covenant, an agreement, a contract with my own being that no matter what, I will come back. I will return to the courage of practice, to the courage of this wee girl with open arms and strong little legs, certain in the eyes of her mother, in the space that holds us and the breath that supports us moment by moment. From that day to this, I do. The gong sounded to end the session and I moved my foot.

{ 3 }

Being Human

We acquire our form within a womb. We are the result of a union of parts that sets our human form into motion. The frame, the stage, the particulars are myriad and shifting, the subject of intense speculation and discourse, the cause of inconceivable bloodshed and violence brought forth by origin myths and our most fervent loyalty to beliefs. Our longing is for a pure and unchallenged explanation for the inexplicable and chaotic display from which we rise and gather cellular energy, bit by bit, until we emerge from an origin story of our own dark sea where we transform from space and mystery. We are pressed and squeezed with wild urgency that will not be stopped until we arrive into the air with the primacy of a reckoning. We begin with that first breath when the diaphragm expands for the first time, and we draw the old world newly in and forever after in our fleshy form.

Where we originated and what we brought and bring, what we carry, all that we offer is with us when we arrive in the midst of a web that clings to us from that first inhalation. We are swaddled, nursed, heralded, and cast out to die, yet still we come into the stories, patterns, and textures of the web that is spun across time - a great adornment of moments and days, an emergence into and release from, the sounds of names repeated that resonate in space as histories, as liturgies, as grudges, as the breath that is the barbaric yawp, laughter, and song. We arrive in the midst of stories in mid-telling. We arrive in the mess and muck of a world that presses and coats and douses and steeps and kneads and plunges us into a current of being, and there we are in the thrall of the humans from whom we have come, and if not those, then some others cross our path and a story is told - a story of logic and madness that we absorb with the senses, infinite details that we gather and label as me and mine and ours. The great union of our arrival is chipped into the jagged falsity of separate truths, that we could possibly be more or less than a compelling and complex display that rises and falls as we open our lungs in the shared space of being again and again and again until the end.

After we arrive as babies, we absorb stories with our highly sensitive being, our physical, energetic, and psychological interplays that receive and share and interpret experience and adjust to situations at hand, forming new patterns from the old, variations on a theme, the repetitions of vibrations that are simply set upon us from birth as part of our path for no particular reason, beyond the myths of karma or divine plan. The patterns that fall upon us are brilliant .They fit to our form and ride in the fertile ground of our hearts to flourish as our own to be traced and tasted. We misperceive and experience a simple misunderstanding when we go off the tracks, away from our own experience and believe in the experience of another more than our own, simply because we do not yet know how human stories flow. We show up on a planet that spins in outer space and is molten at the core . We come into a system of humans that disorients us and we do not learn the essential truths of being a body that seems solid but is mostly space, is resonant, endlessly creative and sensitive. But we can learn.

We have the tools at hand to manifest fully with dignity, brilliance and humor. We can choose the shared lineage of wisdom that is available to us. We can learn the practices that support our journey as a living being, as a form in constant change with unlimited possibility for communication, as the breath moves in and out, now and now and now.

… { 4 }

Longing

I travel to the Scottish isle of Iona to write and to walk. The landscape and the seascape mirror my interior weather. The wind carries a delicate mist that sings a sweet and lonely tune - an ancient cadence carried in rivulets through the heather and stone, in the expansive frame of sky, and in the reaching stretch of sea. When the cracked heart finds shelter, it opens, broadens, and resonates in every cell and becomes the pervasive sky. The cracks are pathways of slow motion. The heart reaches in recognition, without effort, across the smooth beach of stones.

My compact self is undone, comes apart, does not know and has no plan, just opens without a desire or intent or will; and the water blooms; the stones flow; and I am not separate, defined only by the pulse that knows its kin. This place is all that I ever wanted to become. This mist is a truth known only by the gracious ache that rises and spreads and fills and empties and lifts. This is possible: our longing is as simple as the space that is.

We can cherish our broken hearts. We can learn to feel our textures and patterns as in a beloved, with patience and a curiosity for detail. This is different from trying to fix our selves or to make our selves better. We can learn the contours of our own experience right now. We do not have to wait until some point in the future when we are better or when the list has been completed. We can become intimate with exactly where we are on this journey in time. We don't have to be good enough. We can just be.

{ 5 }

Waking Up

As human beings, we encounter difficulty. Perhaps the difficulty is in the form of the people around us or perhaps the situation that we are born into. Possibly we carry patterns of thought or behavior in our heart and head and engage in ways that do not support us and could be shed. This is so normal and is inevitable. Often we create covers with additional layers of thought or behavior. We craft and wear masks to bury our grief, our fear, our anxiety. Our covers become a thick sludge in our lives. We pin ourselves beneath the weight of our own hiding, and we do not know how to come out into the world. We don't remember how to tell the truth. We don't know what the truth feels like. But all is not lost.

A fresh and sparkling clarity is available to us. We can open the window of experience and feel the cold air. We can feel our claustrophobia and fear. We can feel the dullness and the stupefaction that we've put in place. We can feel our tender heart. We can open the locked door of our rage and disappointment. We can experience our own experience. We can taste the moments of our lives in all their detail. With astonishing simplicity, we can learn to wake up to being a body. We can develop an intimate relationship with our selves. We can develop curiosity for our predicament. We can learn how to be. Our shared human wisdom traditions offer simple practices that help us wake up to the brilliance of being as we are at this moment.

{ 6 }

Union

When my parents moved to Birmingham, Alabama in the late 1950's, they rented a small wood frame house. The house was next to a big field that was next to an old farmhouse and barn. Between our rental house and the field was a long row of daffodils. When they bloomed around the time of my birthday, I would lay on the ground close to them. From my spot, I joined a bigger family of flowers and stems and little bugs and drops of water. The sun shined on us as clouds crossed the sky in an unending shift and flow. Here in the field, I was complete, at peace and ease, expansive, surrounded by the smell of daffodils and clover and henbit, wild plantain and daisies as a world of busy insects climbed and flew, hopped and explored with impossibly tiny antennae. The thrum of probing bees going from place to place filled me. In the high trees surrounding my spot in the field the birds crossed my line of vision from time to time. I was warm and safe, and my mother was near and all was well. This was all that I knew.

Later, when I felt torn apart and bewildered, not sure what to do or how to stop making choices that hurt me, I thought back to that big field and those daffodils, to the feeling of union that characterized those moments in the grass.

I love bees and beetles and roly poly's. What a joy to open the rich soil and to discover the life within, the worms and their wiggling gift to the planet as they process their way through the world. I thought deeply about slugs for a year. The slick slug and her tail's trail of mucilage, the surprise of a slug beneath a bare foot or between the toes on a summer night. Slugs devour an enormous amount of garbage. That's right. Slugs are unnoticed allies. This is true for so much in our lives. We prefer to pledge allegiance to the closed loop of our thinking mind of judgments and opinions rather than open to the actual details of the world around us, including our own being.

THE PRACTICE OF BEING

In union we inhabit ourselves. We open to the reality of our physical body. We feel our embodiment, the details of flesh and bone. Our own possibility is so obvious and present, but we often skip past when we could simply open to our body breathing as a starting point. We can feel the space, take a seat, extend the spine, and relax. We can claim our dignity and dwell there.

… { 7 }

The Path

How do we make a path for our longing, our anguish, and our rage to become our healing? I was driving my truck and my nine-year-old son Edward sat beside me. I told him that I could feel myself changing because of my practice. I felt less angry. I asked him what he thought. Could he tell a difference in me? He leaned toward me and put a friendly hand on my shoulder. "Mom" he said. "That's great. Keep practicing!"

In simplest terms, we develop practice as a path, and we keep practicing. Practice is something that we choose to do repeatedly. We create a space in our lives. We put the practice in our schedule. We schedule our time. We explore different types of practice. We see what works in our lives.

My own experience is that the most crucial component of a practice is to show up. Early in my practice, I wanted to be perfect so badly that my only choice was to flee from the dictates of the part of me that demanded perfection or nothing. Actually, this internal dictator was not mine but came from that web of story that covered me when I was born. Over time, as I showed up for the practice again and again, I saw the power of my longing. I understood and appreciated my willingness and commitment to come back to practice and repeat, practice and repeat.

When I first received formal meditation instruction, I was awkward. My mind was wild and bubbly. I didn't want to be angry and miserable anymore. Although psychotherapy helped me to understand the roots, my rage was oppressive and dominated many of my interactions. Rage was one of my well-travelled mental ruts. I wanted to discover a new path. I wanted to to set down the anger that I'd done such a nice job perfecting. I wanted peace, and joy.

The simplicity of the ancient practice of training the mind to follow the breath is helpful. The untrained mind is wild and rebels. Once we tell our mind to feel the breath in the body, the mind kicks and bucks and races around and around. However, with repetition, the mind begins to settle and follows the instruction.

THE PRACTICE OF BEING

I understood that the little girl learning to walk, heading for the arms of her beautiful mother came into clarity because of the space that my practice allowed me to explore. Not only did I learn that rage was a pattern I'd been wearing and could shed, I learned that joy and curiosity are foundational, available to explore and to share. Through practice, a new path is formed.

{ 8 }

Awareness

Awareness is the energy of life that manifests in all beings, in the molecules, the building blocks, the chaos and random motion beyond understanding and yet part of the rise and fall of being. In this way, the practice of activating our self-existing awareness is as normal as learning to throw a ball or to shoot an arrow or to thread a needle. We train our minds to follow instruction so that when we ask it to rest in awareness, that's what happens. The practice of awareness trains us to stay, to dwell in self-existing awareness, to be present for our own experience, to feel the power of our living. We are directly connected to the earth's molten core, to the stars in the galaxies, to the spinning force of the tornado. We are the scorched earth and the new green of a field. We are stones and streams, and we are also flesh. We are we. Each is all, and all is here, spinning in outer space, each with a unique consciousness but none separate.

Separateness is one of the great human misunderstandings. We share an awareness that is the essence of all being. Even stones and steel hold an awareness that is this core. When we train in opening to our connectedness, we can begin to notice that our separateness is an idea, a feeling that has no real basis although we do have a sense of physical boundaries within the physical body that leads us in the direction of feeling separate. Within some cultures, this separation is nurtured and encouraged and results in deep isolation and loneliness. The feeling of being alone can dominate and contribute to challenging issues, such as mental and physical health problems. When we nurture and develop our awareness, we come to grasp the true connectedness of everything. We are then able to communicate with the world in a new and expansive way. The world is in a constant state of communication, and that includes us but is not limited to or defined by us.

If we are cloistered in our own mind, if the mind secludes us rather than including or connecting us, we miss out on the intense power of life and the possibility of deep connection. Although this connection may seem to be primarily with other humans, it is with all beings. The reality of our connectedness simply is. Through awareness practice, we can discover, uncover, revel in, feel supported by, and be in communication with our own physical being as part of a broader world.

To inhabit the awareness of our own being is a totally different experience of life. For example, I grew up in a community with much praise for an examined life. To examine is to look at carefully. But there's more. There's the possibility of expanding our awareness so that we experience an immersion of being. We no longer have to chase thoughts or diversions. We can be, and we can become. Awareness is a naturally occurring state that can be practiced and nurtured. With practice we discover that there is only awareness.

How do we begin this journey? We start with a simple practice of working with the breath. This practice begins to train the mind to settle down so that we can move into the awareness that is what we are. In the process, we discover that breath work is a stabilizing practice that supports our journey in powerful ways.

{ 9 }

Breath

The average person breathes around 25,000 times per day. Yet we often ignore the process completely unless the process becomes a struggle. What could be a more pure expression of our existence as beings than our breathing? We draw in air from the space around and outside of us, and once in our body, nutrients are processed and the rest releases to support other beings. Although we may at times feel isolated and alone, we are in reality in deep relationship with everything that is, and much nurturance is available for us when we learn to wake up to the presence of breath as our life. We can dwell there without trouble or fear. We can simply breath as a profound state of being. We can rest in being a body breathing.

With practice then, we learn to open to and rest in the self-existing awareness of the breath and of breathing. Our wild and untrained minds prefer to roam and bubble without restraint, and we often take this mind as being who and what we are. Yet this is not correct. Our minds require training so that we can open to the depth and expanse of being. Each breath offers an opportunity for our transformation.

Becoming aware of our breath is an ancient practice that remains available and workable as a means of training the mind. We train the mind so that we can move away from the stories that we don't want to keep and towards the hopes, dreams, and goals that we do want to include. We train the mind so that we can inhabit and explore our own being with the space to sort out what's what. The simple practice of breath helps us to learn that we can examine our own experience with the eyes of awareness, and we can make decisions about our own being. We can say, "Oh, look at how I've always identified with being angry, and that really doesn't resonate, so I'm going to set that down and move on into increasing happiness." We can make this choice, and the practice supports us.

We begin to develop new pathways in our minds and in our lives. The mental ruts that have contained and limited us are filled in and smoothed over with practice. Through the repeated return to the feeling of the breath as it enters the body, we slowly transform. We create a new allegiance to the present moment that is always new and always fresh and always now. Like the girl taking her first steps, we can learn to open to the depth and breath of our lives.

What do we practice, and what do we yield? We can sort the practices that we want to continue and what we want to set down. We all have a practice of some sort, maybe the ritual of making coffee, or grooming a dog, or toxic drug use. It's important for us to begin to see our own wisdom as part of our shared wisdom as beings. In this way we learn that training the mind and expanding our awareness is natural for us and is not a concoction emanating from the power of a teacher, organization, or lineage. Before I started to work with breath practice, I practiced as an artist and writer. I explored the present moment for years through art, interpreting music and sound through drawing, sometimes blindfolded. Automatic writing, improvisational theater, and book making have been and still are a few of the forms of my practice.

The heart of the practice is to place our attention on the feeling of the breath as it comes into and out of the nostrils. Then once we notice that we are no longer aware of the feeling of the breath in the nostrils, we go back to the feeling of the breath in the nostrils.

The instruction is as simple as an instruction can be. Do it. We will eventually notice when we have strayed. Do it again. In choosing to follow the breath, we become explorers, not sure what we will encounter. The familiar stories and emotional patterns that claim our attention with great tenacity will shift. This is the challenge of the practice. Over time we notice more. We appreciate more. We deepen.

{ 10 }

Being the Body

We see the images of the calm sage sitting cross-legged on a lotus leaf, eyes closed, hands in a gesture of peace and calm. We might say that practice is supposed to be great, but it's not possible for us to try because we can't sit still. The fact is that the image and the story narrative can be informative as well as discarded. We can come to the practice just as we are. Sitting still is not the point.

We begin the practice in a sitting posture in a chair, lying down, standing up. In the beginning, the main point is to notice the breath in the nostrils as the air moves into the body from the outside and then to notice the feeling as the air leaves the nostrils. With the next inhalation, the attention stays on the feeling of the air entering into the nostrils.

Within this frame of the in-breath and the out-breath, everything happens, and we discover that there is enough space for everything, including us with all of our foibles and neuroses. In the practice of placing our attention on the feeling of air that we draw into and press out of the nostrils, we develop an intimate relationship with ourselves that excludes nothing.

Simply we begin, as we are, not as we wish we were or think that we could be some day down the road when it's different, and we've succeeded in fixing ourselves and crafting a perfect mirage by sheer will. No, that's not what this is about. This is about the details of right now as they unfold. Our natural awareness notices detail. Usually this awareness is dominated or overshadowed by a continual onslaught of thoughts, feelings, and opinions in a rapid and shifting flow. This thinking mind is so prevalent and insistent that we come to think of its motion as our self, as "I". It turns out that there is much more to us than our thinking.

So we take a seat or lie down with the intention to place the attention of the mind on the feeling of the breath in the nostrils as it moves in and out. That's the first step.

At some point we notice that the mind has moved away from the feeling of the breath in the nostrils and that the mind is somewhere else. Thoughts could be anywhere really. We make lists, consider urgent matters, fantasize sexually, plot revenge, panic over pain, feel desperate to get up and do something else, tell ourselves that we've failed at the practice, and on and on and on. There is a moment when we notice that we are gone. We come back to the feeling of the breath. Once again we set the attention on the air as it comes into the body and as it leaves the body.

We are desperate to do something, anything other than this (seemingly) dull, repetitive practice. We all experience this. For some, a slight itch behind the ear becomes a matter of tremendous importance, for example. Or we feel that we will perish if we don't check the phone right now. How sweet and funny, really, the way that we want to squirm away from a simple and straightforward instruction. So to begin, we just find a comfortable spot. Then we notice the feeling of the first breath and the next and the next. Light touch. We notice that we've left the instruction, and we start again.

{ 11 }

The Journey of Practice

Practice is exploration that is done with intention in order to learn to live with full presence, agency, and authority. We practice in order to move into the myriad details of the arc of time that is our lives.

Given the age of the universe and the age of this planet Earth, our lives in this body in this iteration and in this time are brief. With practice we can explore the exquisite details of being, as well as the deep purpose of being that emerges from our practice. We can find out for ourselves. We can uncover the shapes and patterns of meaning that emerge through the repetition of practice and over time form a path, a ground in which we can settle into the feeling of our particulars, into our inherent dignity that rises from the expanded awareness of being a body in space. The way to open into self-existing awareness is through practice.

In this work, I offer a single practice that focuses on the breath and breathing. I have worked extensively with the breath and breathing over the expanse of decades. This work will become particular to you through your attention and repeated exploration.

{ 12 }

Practice Instruction

We shift our attention to the feeling of the breath in the body, to the feeling of the body breathing. Then we narrow the attention around the feeling of the air just as it is drawn into the nostrils at the beginning of a breath. We move our attention, our awareness, to the sensation of the breath just as it turns to breath, as our diaphragm expands and pulls the air into the nasal cavity. We are not engaged in thought or analysis of the process. We set the mind with the task of noticing the breath as it enters the nostrils. When the mind gallops away or froths or sets to shouting, as soon as we notice it, we bring our attention back to the feeling of the breath as it moves in the body. And again the mind moves away. When we notice that we are no longer practicing the instruction, we go back to the start, and we start again.

While this practice can be done at any time, anywhere, and in any physical posture, our wild and unruly minds may offer resistance to our practice. In order to support the practice, we can choose a regular time of day, and a location where we can be free of outside distraction as much as possible. We sit in a comfortable position that is conducive to an alert state. Often when we stop our busy minds with practice, we go straight to sleep. Since our intention is to practice, we do need to be awake. Therefore sitting upright is helpful. A cushion, chair, or stool is suggested.

Many instructions for meditation practice offer elaborate and rigid step-by-step details of the practice process. But a more natural and simple process is possible and helps us to discover that the practice is a spacious creative process rather than another thing that we have to perfect or else risk failure. We can explore our lives, and in order to do so, it is helpful to train our minds so that we are not dominated by our thinking, emotions, and judgments. When we follow the breath, we are training the mind to settle down.

We can simply feel the breath as it comes into and out of the body. That is enough. This moment is magical and monumental. This intake, initiated by the expansion of the diaphragm muscle pulls the space - the air, the outer world - into our noses, into the beautiful delivery system that moves the air through the throat and into the lungs where the air is processed and is then expelled as the diaphragm contracts.

How did we come to believe that we were/are separate? The mind refers to itself as a primary attention. The contours of the body and the perimeter of the skin inform the identity of separateness. Indeed, we are not separate as we draw in the air that surrounds and contains not only our own being but all being as we live through the force of the nutrients generated by the myriad forms of being on this planet and in this cosmos. We are here together.

As we work with our minds and gently train the mind to settle down to relax, we are not judging the mind or its content. We are simply participating in a practice that stretches back through time and across space, we can deepen as living beings. We can come to a more detailed and intimate relationship with our own living.

The breath and the body are almost indistinguishable. We settle the mind and open our awareness and follow the breath in its path. When the mind is wild, we can rest at the entrance of the nostrils. When the mind is calm, we can follow the breath in its path as we open the awareness to the ceaseless details of our own experience as living beings. We can rest in the experience of the ribs opening as the lungs expand with the intake of air. We can feel the heart as it circulates the blood that is enriched and invigorated with each breath. We can simply be, with our own authority, informed from the inside, from the details of this moment of being, and this one, and this.

Of course, the mind then jumps in with its dependable chatter and plans and plots and considerations. An old math problem pops up. A memory of an argument arises and we feel it resonate in our chest. A fragment of a song plays on a loop in our head. All of this is the beautiful fodder of our lives and yet, there is so much more that is the reality of our situation as beings, and we miss it because we mistake the mind for our lives.

We can become sovereign. Our story can unfold as our own, inextricably connected to other beings, to the elements to the forces of the universe, to that which we cannot imagine.

Through the simple practice of following the breath again and again, we open to the unbroken, unceasing awareness that is waiting for us to connect and to be.

{ 13 }

Becoming Intimate

Our capacity for intimacy with our own felt sense of being is always possible. We can move into the process of learning more and more about our experience with its details and subtleties. In this way, the idea of intimacy is no longer reserved for a partner but for our own being. As we practice, we encounter the feelings of hope, fear, rage, fantasy, aversion, and scheming again and again. The things that we shun, the thoughts that cause shame, all become familiar over time, and this is how we develop an abiding intimacy with ourselves.

As we feel into our bodies in our practice, we gain a deeper understanding of our experience. We uncover and step into all aspects of our being. We may realize that we would benefit from guides—therapists and teachers—people familiar with some of the challenges of deep process work, who can help us along the way or at various points. Of course, not all guides are right for all people, so a proper vetting is always appropriate. We begin to learn about what we need.

With practice, we notice the same sorts of mental activity again and again, and eventually we become thoroughly familiar with our experience. This is far different from the scheme to be perfect or the self-improvement projects that can be so brutal in our lives. We are talking about coming to the table as we are with all of the muck of our lives, including our problems, phobias, aggressions, and aversions. Everything is included in this journey. The longing to be fully ourselves, to be known and to be seen—this is the process that we can claim for ourselves, for this fleshy reality, for this heart and this mind.

Once upon a time, an image formed in my mind, and a story rose with it. The image was of a cave, a dark cave. My job was to enter this cave even though I was afraid and to explore the cave with all of my senses. I was to become thoroughly intimate with the cave through the texture and shape of the walls, the smells and the sounds, and through the presence of my fear. This is true of our practice. I discovered that my fears were actually based in fears that had been projected upon me as a child and that I am not a fearful person. I continue to work with my experience, as a body moving in a time continuum, as an intellect making connections and discoveries, as a heart that opens and closes with a longing for openness and connection. The dark cave is not other but is a discovery. It is data, beyond labels.

Everything in our lives is workable. We can learn to appreciate our own fear, our own neurosis. We can say, "Oh that rage at my brother, that's an old story and an old wound so dependably present in my life," and we deepen into the details more and more. As our minds settle through practice, we can access our stories, our wounds, and our longings with our senses. We no longer contain dark caves that we fear to enter, but rather we explore our landscape, dark spaces and light. We develop an abiding intimacy with ourselves.

{ 14 }

Mental Weather

One of the most powerful benefits of practice is that we loosen the grip on our minds, and we begin to notice the deeply embedded and ever changing patterns of our minds. We start to notice our mental weather. What we cling to as "I/me/mine" may be a bit different from what we've supposed. We could take a moment right now to ask: "What is my mental weather?" And then simply notice. Are we agitated, cheerful, gloomy, sad, or anxious? Just as the atmospheric weather is moving and changing constantly around the planet, we experience mental weather of the mind. We can learn to notice the weather in ourselves, and as we do, we can see that we don't have to act out against an ever-changing situation. We can learn to observe and to witness rather than simply reacting. We gain insight, and this in one of the most beautiful results of practice. We begin to see both the causes and the conditions of our own lives, and we start to see through the seeming solidity of our state of mind. We begin to see that our mind is pliant and can be more calm, more happy, more caring, and more discerning.

We can consider, for example, a time when we were annoyed or angry for no discernible reason. This happens for many of us from time to time with varying frequency. Perhaps we reacted to our state of mind, our mental weather, by being sharp or hurtful to others. Or perhaps we were plagued by angry thoughts rolling around, filling up the space, crowding out the possibility for joy, for experiencing the ecstatic detail of being, including the pain and the trauma and the boredom and the rage. The fact is that we can come as we are. The mental weather does not need to be sunny in order for us to work with our lives as human beings. We can work with whatever rises and that is a great cause for celebration.

{ 15 }

Wisdom

The practice of working with the breath in the body, of opening to the awareness of the body, of sorting our experience, and determining our purpose comes from our shared and ancient wisdom as humans. I did not make up this information. I have teachers who had teachers who had teachers and back into the stretch of time. Human wisdom traditions point in the same direction to the path of transformation. The myths, beliefs, and rituals can differ, but to a large extent, the purpose is to lead human beings to change, to move away from the confining sense of self and into the power of the connected whole, to source. We are built for reverence, respect and revelry. We are made to witness beauty and to understand that we are connected to the great mystery of source, that we embody the wisdom of the universe.

When we rest in the awareness of the breath in the body and when we notice that we are lost in thought, as we do and as we will, and when we return to the breath, we develop a new allegiance that is not bound by any religion or philosophy. The breath is a vehicle or conduit for our journey. Our journey is an exploration of life in which all our experience is included. We learn to feel everything. This process transforms us, softens us, and heals us.

We benefit from the support and guidance of a practice community, and while we may enjoy and profit from the shared experience and insight of teachers, the role of the exclusive wisdom keeper who controls from the top can lead us away from the direct flavor of source. Each of us carries the seeds of our own unique and personal becoming. In this way, we don't have to accept or reject the religious traditions that abound, although we may choose to reject views that exclude and diminish ourselves or others, including the natural world, that hearken to an "us and them" mentality or power structure. This is always a path that leads us away from the heart of wisdom. Such systems are convenient for creating efficient organizations that manage people, but they cannot and do not lead to our freedom. The path of freedom is our wisdom.

{ 16 }

Choosing to Practice

As I breathe, I feel the rawness of my heart. I am still the little girl connected to the earth and to my mother. I am the mother nursing her baby. I am the woman whose dreams didn't work out. I feel the breath expand in my body. I feel the breath leave my body. Thoughts arise. They are swift and appear in torrents. I want to follow them. At some point, I notice that I am lost in thought. When I notice this, I go back to the feeling of the breath in my body.

Why do I go back to the practice of being the body breathing? It's quite simple. When I practice,

I can simply experience what is. This is a relief. My incessant desire to manipulate my experience generates pain. When I can simply experience the roots of my experience, the roots of my lives, I transform. I heal when I sit with the broken heart and feel my disappointment and grief and rage and fear. With each breath in and each breath out, I connect rather than attempt to flee a situation that I cannot escape. I hold my pain in the open hands of my practice. In the process, I discover that I am not alone. We are here together.

Acknowledgments

Many thanks to my son Edward F. Mostoller for his kindness and encouragement and to my husband Robert E. Heithaus, Sr for his support of my workspaces, my practice, and my silence. I am grateful for the hospitality and of Elisabeth Rosales and cellist Craig Hultgren who supported me in the writing process. I thank Dr Leisha Hultgren for her editorial aid. My good fortune is to encounter and learn with powerful teachers in myriad forms. I offer gratitude that this is so. I bow to you.

Resources

To learn more about Creative Awareness and the work of the Creative Awareness Institute

www.creativeawarenessinstitute.com

Projects include:
- Creative Awareness Practice
- Forest Bathing
- Aging and the Sacred Arc of Time
- Tantric Body Awareness
- Grown Women Are Hairy
- The Contemplative Practice of Writing

About Anne Markham Bailey

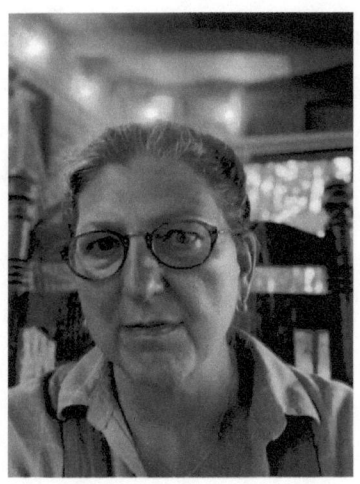

Anne Markham Bailey is a writer based in Birmingham, Alabama. A graduate of Barnard College at Columbia University in New York, Bailey majored in East Asian Studies with a concentration in Chinese language and literature. She holds an MFA in Book Arts and an MA in English, Creative Writing. She has published two books of poems *Cold Stone, White Lily* and

Nancy Marguerite's Chopin, and a children's book, *The Daring Egg*. Her podcast Present Tense produced a 13-part series, "The Fight For Alabama's Last Wild Places" in 2019. She is a meditation teacher with a deep interest in somatic awareness. In 2021 she founded Creative Awareness Institute. To learn more, go to annemarkhambailey.com

The mission of the Institute is to explore and offer projects, programs, and practices that engage creativity, lead us to connect as beings, and build pathways for deep awareness and peace in society.

www.ingramcontent.com/pod-product-compliance
Lightning Source LLC
Chambersburg PA
CBHW020546080526
44583CB00013B/1026